Introduction to the Alkaline Diet:

"Improving Your Health and Well-being with a Plant Based Diet"

J. Ceesay

Legal & Disclaimer

The information contained in this book and its contents is not designed to replace or take the place of any form of medical or professional advice; and is not meant to replace the need for independent medical, financial, legal or other professional advice or services, as may be required. The content and information in this book have been provided for educational and entertainment purposes only.

The content and information contained in this book has been compiled from sources deemed reliable, and it is accurate to the best of the Author's knowledge, information and belief. However, the Author cannot guarantee its accuracy and validity and cannot be held liable for any errors and/or omissions. Further, changes are periodically made to this book as and when needed. Where appropriate and/or necessary, you must consult a professional (including but not limited to your doctor, attorney, financial advisor or such other professional advisor) before using any of the suggested remedies, techniques, or information in this book.

Upon using the contents and information contained in this book, you agree to hold harmless the Author from and against any damages, costs, and expenses, including any legal fees potentially resulting from the application of any of the information provided by this book. This disclaimer

Table Of Contents

Introduction

What Is an Alkaline Diet?

An alkaline diet — also known as the alkaline ash diet, alkaline acid diet, acid ash diet, acid alkaline diet and even sometimes the pH diet — is one that helps balance the blood pH level of the fluids in your body, including your blood and urine. Your pH is partially determined by the mineral density of the foods you eat. All living organisms and life forms on earth depend on maintaining appropriate pH levels, and it's often said that disease and disorder cannot take root in a body that has a balanced pH.

The principles of the acid ash hypothesis help make up the tenets of the alkaline diet. According to research published in Journal of Bone and Mineral Research, "The acid-ash hypothesis posits that protein and grain foods, with a low potassium intake, produce a diet acid load, net acid excretion (NAE), increased urine calcium, and release of calcium from the skeleton, leading to osteoporosis." The alkaline diet aims to prevent this from happening by carefully taking food pH levels into consideration in an attempt to limit dietary acid intake.

Although some experts might not totally agree with this statement, nearly all agree that human life requires a very tightly controlled pH level of the blood of about 7.365–7.4. As Forbe's Magazine puts it, "Our bodies go to extraordinary lengths to maintain safe pH levels." Your pH can range between 7.35 to 7.45 depending on the time of day, your diet, what you last ate and when you last went to the bathroom. If you develop electrolyte imbalances and fre☐uently consume too many acidic foods — aka acid ash foods — your body's changing pH level can result in increased "acidosis."

Wondering what exactly "pH level" even means?

What we call pH is short for the potential of hydrogen. It's a measure of the acidity or alkalinity of our body's fluids and tissues. It's measured on a scale from 0 to 14. The more acidic a solution is, the lower its pH. The more alkaline, the higher the number is. A pH of around 7 is considered neutral, but since the optimal human body tends to be around 7.4, we consider the healthiest pH to be one that's slightly alkaline, and pH levels vary throughout the body, with the stomach being the most acidic region.

Even very tiny alterations in the pH level of various organisms can cause major problems. For example, due to environmental concerns, such as increasing CO_2 deposition, the pH of the ocean has dropped from 8.2 to 8.1 and various life forms living in the ocean have greatly suffered. The pH level is also crucial for growing plants, and therefore it greatly affects the mineral content of the foods we eat. Minerals in the ocean, oil and human body are used as buffers to maintain optimal pH levels, so when acidity rises, minerals fall.

Chapter One

How an Alkaline Diet Works

Here's some background on acid/alkalinity in the human diet, plus key points about how alkaline diets can be beneficial:

Researchers believe that when it comes to the total acid load of the human diet, "there have been considerable changes from hunter gather civilizations to the present." Following the agricultural revolution and then mass industrialization of our food supply over the last 200 years, the food we eat has significantly less potassium, magnesium and chloride, along with more sodium, compared to diets of the past.

Normally, the kidneys maintain our electrolyte levels (those of calcium, magnesium, potassium and sodium). When we're exposed to overly acidic substances, these electrolytes are used to combat acidity.

According to the Journal of Environmental Health review mentioned earlier, the ratio of potassium to sodium in most people's diets has changed dramatically. Potassium used to outnumber sodium by 10:1, however now the ratio has dropped to 1:3. People eating a "Standard American Diet" now consume three times as much sodium as potassium on average!

Many children and adults today consume a high-sodium diet that's very low in not only magnesium and potassium, but also antioxidants, fiber and essential vitamins. On top of that, the typical Western diet is high in refined fats, simple sugars, sodium and chloride.

All of these changes to the human diet have resulted in increased "metabolic acidosis." In other words, the pH levels of many people's bodies are no longer optimal. On top of this, many are suffering from low nutrient intake and problems such as potassium and magnesium deficiency.

This accelerates the aging process, causes gradual loss of organ functions, and degenerates tissue and bone mass. High degrees of acidity force our bodies to rob minerals from the bones, cells, organs and tissues.

What it Does

1. Protects Bone Density and Muscle Mass

Your intake of minerals plays an important role in the development and maintenance of bone structures. Research shows that the more alkalizing fruits and vegetables someone eats, the better protection that person might have from experiencing decreased bone strength and muscle wasting as they age, known as sarcopenia.

An alkaline diet can help balance ratios of minerals that are important for building bones and maintaining lean muscle mass, including calcium, magnesium and phosphate. Alkaline diets also help improve production of growth hormones and vitamin D absorption, which further protects bones in addition to mitigating many other chronic diseases.

2. Lowers Risk for Hypertension and Stroke

One of the anti-aging effects of an alkaline diet is that it decreases inflammation and causes an increase in growth hormone production. This has been shown to improve cardiovascular health and offer protection against common problems like high cholesterol, hypertension (high blood pressure), kidney stones, stroke and even memory loss.

3. Lowers Chronic Pain and Inflammation

Studies have found a connection between an alkaline diet and reduced levels of chronic pain. Chronic acidosis has been found to contribute to chronic back pain, headaches, muscle spasms, menstrual symptoms, inflammation and joint pain.

One study conducted by the Society for Minerals and Trace Elements in Germany found that when patients with chronic back pain were given an alkaline supplement daily for four weeks, 76 of 82 patients reported significant decreases in pain as measured by the Arhus low back pain rating scale.

4. Boosts Vitamin Absorption and Prevents Magnesium Deficiency

An increase in magnesium is required for the function of hundreds of enzyme systems and bodily processes. Many people are deficient in magnesium and as a result experience heart complications, muscle pains, headaches, sleep troubles and anxiety. Available magnesium is also required to activate vitamin D and prevent vitamin D deficiency, which is important for overall immune and endocrine functioning.

5. Helps Improve Immune Function and Cancer Protection

When cells lack enough minerals to properly dispose of waste or oxygenate the body fully, the whole body suffers. Vitamin absorption is compromised by mineral loss, while toxins and pathogens accumulate in the body and weaken the immune system.

Research published in the British Journal of Radiology showed that cancerous cell death (apoptosis) was more likely to occur in an alkaline body. Cancer prevention is believed to be associated with an alkaline shift in pH due to an alteration in electric charges and the release of basic components of proteins. Alkalinity can help decrease inflammation and the risk for diseases like cancer — plus an alkaline diet has been shown to be more beneficial for some chemotherapeutic agents that require a higher pH to work appropriately.

6. Can Help You Maintain a Healthy Weight

Limiting consumption of acid-forming foods and eating more alkaline-forming foods can protect your body from obesity by decreasing leptin levels and inflammation, which affects your hunger and fat-burning abilities. Since alkaline-forming foods are anti-inflammatory foods, consuming an alkaline diet gives your body a chance to achieve normal leptin levels and feel satisfied from eating the amount of calories you really need.

Chapter Two

How to Eat an Alkaline Diet

This chapter will teach you on how you can eat Alkaline Diet. Here are some key tips for following an alkaline diet:

Whenever possible, try to buy organic alkaline foods. Experts feel that one important consideration in regard to eating an alkaline diet is to become knowledgeable about what type of soil your produce was grown in — since fruits and vegetables that are grown in organic, mineral-dense soil tend to be more alkalizing. Research shows that the type of soil that plants are grown in can significantly influence their vitamin and mineral content, which means not all "alkaline foods" are created e□ually.

The ideal pH of soil for the best overall availability of essential nutrients in plants is between 6 and 7. Acidic soils below a pH of 6 may have reduced calcium and magnesium, and soil above a pH of 7 may result in chemically unavailable iron, manganese, copper and zinc. Soil that's well-rotated, organically sustained and exposed to wildlife/grazing cattle tends to be the healthiest.

If you're curious to know your pH level before implementing the tips below, you can test your pH by purchasing strips at your local health food store or pharmacy. You can measure your pH with saliva or urine. Your second urination of the morning will give you the best results. You compare the colors on your test strip to a chart that comes with your test strip kit. During the day, the best time to test your pH is one hour before a meal and two hours after a meal. If you test with your saliva, you want to try to stay between 6.8 and 7.2.

Best Alkaline Foods:

Fresh fruits and vegetables promote alkalinity the most. Some of the top picks include mushrooms, citrus, dates, raisins, spinach, grapefruit, tomatoes, avocado, summer black radish, alfalfa grass, barley grass, cucumber, kale, jicama, wheat grass, broccoli, oregano, garlic, ginger, green beans, endive, cabbage, celery, red beet, watermelon, figs and ripe bananas.

All raw foods: Ideally try to consume a good portion of your produce raw. Uncooked fruits and vegetables are said to be biogenic or "life-giving." Cooking foods depletes alkalizing minerals. Increase your intake of raw foods, and try juicing or lightly steaming fruits and vegetables.

Plant proteins: Almonds, navy beans, lima beans and most other beans are good choices.

Alkaline water: Alkaline water has a pH of 9 to 11. Distilled water is just fine to drink. Water filtered with a reverse osmosis filter is slightly acidic, but it's still a far better option than tap water or purified bottled water. Adding pH drops, lemon or lime, or baking soda to your water can also boosts its alkalinity.

Green drinks: Drinks made from green vegetables and grasses in powder form are loaded with alkaline-forming foods and chlorophyll. Chlorophyll is structurally similar to our own blood and helps alkalize the blood.

Other foods to eat on an alkaline diet include sprouts, wheatgrass, kamut, fermented soy like natto or tempeh, and seeds.

Anti-Alkaline Foods and Habits:

Foods that contribute most to acidity include:

High-sodium foods: Processed foods contain tons of sodium chloride — table salt — which constricts blood vessels and creates acidity.

Cold cuts and conventional meats

Processed cereals (such as corn flakes)

Eggs

Caffeinated drinks and alcohol

Oats and whole wheat products: All grains, whole or not, create acidity in the body. Americans ingest most of their plant food quota in the form of processed corn or wheat.

Milk: Calcium-rich dairy products cause some of the highest rates of osteoporosis. That's because they create acidity in the body! When your bloodstream becomes too acidic, it will steal calcium (a more alkaline substance) from the bones to try to balance out the pH level. So the best way to prevent osteoporosis is to eat lots of alkaline green leafy veggies!

Peanuts and walnuts

Pasta, rice, bread and packaged grain products

What other kinds of habits can cause acidity in your body? The biggest offenders include:

Alcohol and drug use

High caffeine intake

Antibiotic overuse

Artificial sweeteners

Chronic stress

Declining nutrient levels in foods due to industrial farming

Low levels of fiber in the diet

Lack of exercise

Excess animal meats in the diet (from non-grass-fed sources)

Excess hormones from foods, health and beauty products, and plastics

Exposure to chemicals and radiation from household cleansers, building materials, computers, cell phones and microwaves

Food coloring and preservatives

Over-exercise

Pesticides and herbicides

Pollution

Poor chewing and eating habits

Processed and refined foods

Shallow breathing

Alkaline Diet vs. Paleo Diet

The Paleo diet and alkaline diet have many things in common and a lot of the same benefits, such as lowered risk for nutrient deficiencies, reduced inflammation levels, better digestion, weight loss or management, and so on.

Some things that the two have in common include eliminating added sugars, reducing intake of pro-inflammatory omega-6 fatty acids, eliminating grains and processed carbs, decreasing or eliminating dairy/milk intake, and increasing intake of fruits and veggies.

However, there are several important things to consider if you plan to follow the Paleo diet. The

Paleo diet eliminates all dairy products, including yogurt and kefir, which can be valuable sources of probiotics and minerals for many people — plus the Paleo diet doesn't always emphasize eating organic foods or grass-fed/free-range meat (and in moderation/limited ⬜uantities).

Additionally, the Paleo diet tends to include lots of meat, pork and shellfish, which have their own drawbacks.

Eating too many animal sources of protein in general can actually contribute to acidity, not alkalinity. Beef, chicken, cold cuts, shellfish and pork can contribute to sulfuric acid buildup in the blood as amino acids are broken down. Try to obtain the best ⬜uality animal products you can, and vary your intake of protein foods to balance your pH level best.

Approaches

Choosing an alkaline lifestyle can be done ⬜uite easily. As a rule of thumb, choosing 70 percent alkaline foods (veggies and legumes) and 30 percent acidic foods (meat and carbs) is the way to go, but any little change makes a difference. Here are some key steps to living an alkaline lifestyle:

1. Eat green

Fresh fruit, vegetables, roots, nuts and legumes are alkalizing to the body, so increase the amount of fruits and vegetables you eat. Aim to have some at every meal and make vegetables the focus rather than meat or grains. Reach for dark or green vegetables such as beetroot, avocado, broccoli, spinach, kale, peas, beans and cucumber.

2. Reduce acidic foods

You don't have to cut them out altogether but try and limit your intake of meats, eggs, refined sugars, white flour and dairy.

3. Limit alcohol consumption

Most alcoholic beverages have a high sugar content and are highly acidic. You don't have to cut it out altogether if you enjoy the occasional beer or glass of wine, but be aware of what you are drinking. (Click here for more on the benefits of cutting back on alcohol.)

4. Drink alkaline water

Drinking water is vital to our health and most of us don't drink enough to begin with. Hydrate yourself with eight to 10 large glasses of alkaline water per day.

Most tap water has a pH of 6.5 to 7, while alkaline water has a pH of 9, making it better at rebalancing the acid-alkaline levels in your body. Alkaline water molecules are also smaller than those of tap water. This means they permeate your body more thoroughly and leave you more hydrated than regular water.

5. Choose natural energy-boost drinks

Forget sugar- and caffeine-laden energy drinks. Choose natural, alkalizing energy drinks such as peppermint tea, yerba maté tea, lemon water or a green powder supplement that can cleanse the digestive system, stimulate your metabolism and buffer excess acids. (Click here for a great alkalizing smoothie recipe.)

6. Break a sweat

Exercise for at least 30 minutes three to five times a week. Among its many benefits, exercise helps counteract acidity in our bodies and sweat gives acid another pathway out of the body. Plus, it helps to oxygenate and alkalize your blood.

7. Seek balance

Stress contributes to acid build-up so find ways to de-stress. Meditation, yoga, deep breathing and long walks are all great ways to de-stress and reduce acid levels.

In addition to helping you losing weight, the alkaline diet is also able to give you more energy, lower your risk of type 2 diabetes, kidney problems and other chronic diseases, reduce joint pain and lactic-acid build up (leg cramps), give you clearer skin and improve your bone health. If you decide to go alkaline, start by making incremental changes to your diet. You're most likely to succeed if you take on change gradually. Every little change is one more step toward better long term health.

Chapter Three

A 7-Day Alkaline Meal Plan

Going alkaline doesn't mean cutting foods completely out of your diet, so let's not focus on elimination. Rather, think of all the delicious, fresh and healthy foods you can eat to promote alkalinity. To help you through it, this is a seven-day meal plan with alkaline recipes (using ingredients you already probably work with all the time) to help get you started. Prepare to feel more energized and pain-free in no time!

DAY ONE

Breakfast: Strawberry Coco Chia Quinoa Breakfast

Ingredients:

- ✓ *1 cup cooked ⬜uinoa*
- ✓ *5 tbsp. chia seeds*
- ✓ *1 ½ cup almond, coconut or hemp milk*
- ✓ *½ cup ⬜uartered strawberries + 4 sliced strawberries*
- ✓ *2 pitted date*
- ✓ *2 tbsp. almond pieces*
- ✓ *2 tbsp. unsweetened shredded coconut flakes*

Directions:

The night before, cook ⬜uinoa and prepare strawberry chia by combining the strawberries, almond milk, and 2 dates in a blender and pureeing until smooth. Pour the mixture into a jar and add chia seeds. Mix well until all chia seeds are covered with the liquid. Cover with lid and refrigerate overnight. In the morning, place chia seeds in bowl, add the ⬜uinoa and strawberry slices, almonds, and shredded coconut and enjoy!

Lunch: Sweet and Savory Salad

Ingredients:

- ✓ *1 large head of butter lettuce*
- ✓ *½ cucumber, sliced*
- ✓ *1 pomegranate, seeded or 1/3 cup seeds*
- ✓ *1 avocado, cubed*
- ✓ *¼ cup shelled pistachios, chopped*

Dressing Ingredients:

- ✓ *¼ cup apple cider vinegar*
- ✓ *½ cup extra virgin olive oil*
- ✓ *1 garlic clove, minced*

Directions:

Hand tear the butter lettuce into a salad bowl. Add the rest of the ingredients and toss with the salad dressing.

DAY TWO

Breakfast: Non-Dairy Apple Parfait

Ingredients:

- ✓ *½ cup soaked raw cashews (soak 20 mins-1 hour)*
- ✓ *½ cup unsweetened almond or coconut milk*
- ✓ *½ tsp. vanilla*
- ✓ *1 cup chopped apple*
- ✓ *1/3 cup rolled gluten-free oats, uncooked*
- ✓ *1 tbsp. hemp seeds*

Directions:

Combine cashews, almond milk, and vanilla in a blender and blend until smooth. Layer ingredients in a small cup: heaping spoon of cashew cream, spoonful of apples, top with oats and hemp seeds and enjoy!

Lunch: Savory Avocado Wrap

Ingredients:

- ✓ 1 butter lettuce or collard leaf bunch
- ✓ ½ haas avocado
- ✓ 1 tsp. chopped basil
- ✓ Small handful of spinach
- ✓ 1 tsp. cilantro, chopped
- ✓ ¼ red onion, diced
- ✓ 1 tomato, sliced or chopped
- ✓ Sea salt & pepper

Directions:

Spread avocado onto leaf and sprinkle with basil, cilantro, red onion, tomato, salt and pepper and add spinach. Fold in half and enjoy!

DAY THREE

Breakfast: Almond Butter Crunch Berry Smoothie

Ingredients:

- ✓ 2 cups fresh spinach
- ✓ 2 cups almond milk, unsweetened
- ✓ 1 cup of any of the following (frozen mixed berries, strawberries or grapes)
- ✓ 1 banana (peeled and frozen)
- ✓ 4 tbsp. raw almond butter
- ✓ 1 tbsp. chia

Directions:

Blend spinach and almond milk first. Then add remaining ingredients except chia, and blend. Add chia once all is smooth – then blend on a very low speed to mix. If you don't have a variable speed blender, mix chia in with the rest of the ingredients by hand. Let sit for a few minutes for the chia seeds to expand, then enjoy.

Lunch: Kale Pesto Pasta

Ingredients:

- ✓ 1 bunch kale
- ✓ 2 cups fresh basil
- ✓ 1/4 cup extra virgin olive oil
- ✓ 1/2 cup walnuts
- ✓ 2 limes, fresh s□ueezed
- ✓ Sea salt and pepper
- ✓ 1 zucchini, noodled (spiralizer)
- ✓ Optional: garnish with sliced asparagus, spinach leaves, and tomato

Directions:

The night before, soak walnuts to improve absorption. Put all ingredients in a blender or food processor, and blend until you get a cream consistency. Add to zucchini noodles and enjoy!

DAY FOUR

Breakfast: Apple and Almond Butter Oats

Ingredients:

- ✓ *2 cups gluten-free oats*
- ✓ *1 ½ cups coconut milk*
- ✓ *1/3 cup raw almond butter*
- ✓ *1 cup grated green apple*
- ✓ *1 tsp. cinnamon*

Directions:

Add the oats, coconut milk and almond butter into a bowl and mix well. Stir in the grated apple; cover the bowl with a lid or plastic wrap and place in the refrigerator. Refrigerate overnight. If the oats get too thick, add some coconut milk to them. Garnish with cinnamon powder.

Lunch: Green Goddess Bowl with Avocado Cumin Dressing

Ingredients for avocado cumin dressing:

- ✓ *1 avocado*
- ✓ *1 tbsp. cumin powder*

- ✓ 2 limes, fresh s☐ueezed
- ✓ 1 cup filtered water
- ✓ ¼ tsp. sea salt
- ✓ 1 tbsp. extra virgin olive oil
- ✓ dash cayenne pepper
- ✓ Optional: ¼ tsp. smoked paprika
- ✓ Ingredients for Tahini Lemon Dressing:
- ✓ ¼ cup tahini (sesame butter)
- ✓ ½ cup filtered water (more if you desire thinner, less for thicker)
- ✓ ½ lemon, fresh s☐ueezed
- ✓ 1 clove minced garlic
- ✓ ¾ tsp. sea salt (Celtic grey, Himalayan, Redmond Real Salt)
- ✓ 1 tbsp. extra virgin olive oil
- ✓ Black pepper to taste

Ingredients for salad:

- ✓ 3 cups kale, chopped
- ✓ ½ cup broccoli florets, chopped
- ✓ ½ zucchini (make noodles with spiralizer)
- ✓ ½ cup kelp noodles, soaked and drained
- ✓ 1/3 cup cherry tomatoes, halved
- ✓ 2 tbsp. hemp seeds

Directions:

Lightly steam kale and broccoli (flash steam for 4 minutes), set aside. Mix zucchini noodles and kelp noodles and toss with a generous serving of smoked avocado cumin dressing. Add cherry tomatoes and toss again. Plate the steamed kale and broccoli and drizzle them with lemon tahini dressing. Top kale and broccoli with the dressed noodles and tomatoes and sprinkle the whole dish with hemp seeds.

DAY FIVE

Breakfast: Berry Good Spinach Power Smoothie

Ingredients:

- ✓ *2 cups fresh spinach*
- ✓ *2 cups unsweetened almond milk*
- ✓ *1 cup frozen mixed berries*
- ✓ *1 frozen banana*
- ✓ *1 tbsp. coconut oil*
- ✓ *½ tsp. cinnamon*
- ✓ *2 tbsp. raw almond butter*

Directions:

Blend spinach and almond milk first, then add remaining ingredients and blend.

Lunch: Quinoa Burrito Bowl (Get Off Your Acid 7-Day Cleanse FAVORITE!)

Ingredients:

- ✓ 1 cup quinoa (or brown rice)
- ✓ 2 15-oz cans of black or adzuki beans
- ✓ 4 green onions (scallions), sliced
- ✓ 2 limes, fresh juiced
- ✓ 4 garlic cloves, minced
- ✓ 1 heaping tsp. cumin
- ✓ 2 avocados, sliced
- ✓ small handful of cilantro, chopped

Directions:

Cook ᐧuinoa or rice. While cooking, warm beans over low heat. Stir in onions, lime juice, garlic and cumin and let flavors combine for 10-15 minutes. When ᐧuinoa is done cooking, divide into individual serving bowls. Top with beans, avocado and cilantro.

DAY SIX

Breakfast: Quinoa Morning Porridge

Ingredients:

- ✓ ½ cup rinsed ᐧuinoa
- ✓ 1 15 oz. can of coconut milk
- ✓ 1 tsp. cinnamon
- ✓ 1 tsp. chia seeds
- ✓ 1 tsp. hemp seeds

Directions:

Combine all ingredients except hemp seeds and simmer for 10-15 minutes until liuid is absorbed. Sprinkle with hemp seeds.

Lunch: Thai Quinoa Salad

Ingredients for dressing:

- ✓ *1 tbsp. sesame seeds*
- ✓ *1 tsp. chopped garlic*
- ✓ *1 tsp. lemon, fresh juiced*
- ✓ *3 tsp. apple cider vinegar*
- ✓ *2 tsp. tamari, gluten-free*
- ✓ *¼ cup tahini (sesame butter)*
- ✓ *1 pitted date*
- ✓ *½ tsp. salt*
- ✓ *½ tsp. toasted sesame oil*

Ingredients for salad:

- ✓ *1 cup of uinoa, steamed*
- ✓ *1 large handful of arugula*
- ✓ *1 tomato, sliced*
- ✓ *¼ red onion, diced*

Directions:

In a small blender, add the following: ¼ cup + 2 tbsp. filtered water, then the rest of ingredients. Blend. Steam 1 cup of quinoa in a steamer or rice cooker, then set aside. Combine, quinoa, arugula, sliced tomatoes, diced red onion, onto a serving plate or bowl, add Thai dressing, and hand mix with a spoon and serve.

DAY SEVEN

Breakfast: Alkamind Warrior Chia Breakfast

Ingredients:

- ✓ 1 cup unsweetened almond or coconut milk
- ✓ 4 tbsp. of chia seeds
- ✓ ½ tsp. vanilla
- ✓ ½ tsp. cinnamon
- ✓ 1 tbsp. unsweetened shredded coconut flakes
- ✓ ¼ cup chopped nuts (almonds, cashews or hemp seeds)

Directions:

The night before, combine milk and chia seeds in a mason jar. Add vanilla, cinnamon and chopped nuts. Cover with lid and shake the mixture until it's combined. Refrigerate overnight. The next morning, shake or stir the mixture and divide into

2-3 bowls. Top with optional fresh fruit, coconut shreds or more chopped nuts.

Lunch: *Asian Sesame Dressing and Noodles*

Ingredients for dressing:

- ✓ *2 tbsp. tahini (sesame butter)*
- ✓ *2 tsp. tamari (gluten-free)*
- ✓ *½ tsp. liquid coconut nectar (Coconut Secrets brand)*
- ✓ *½ tsp. lemon, fresh squeezed 1 clove garlic, minced*

Ingredients for noodle salad:

- ✓ *1 scallion, chopped*
- ✓ *1 tbsp. raw sesame seeds (topping)*
- ✓ *Optional: sliced red bell pepper and/or carrot*

Directions:

Choose one of the following for noodles: Kelp Noodles (1 bag) or 1 Zucchini (use spiralizer or vegetable peeler)

In a mixing bowl, combine all the dressing ingredients and thoroughly mix with a spoon. Make your zucchini noodles with a spiralizer or, if using kelp noodles, place in warm water for 10 minutes to rinse off the liquid they are packaged with, allowing them to separate and soften. Add the Asian Sesame dressing to the noodles and scallions, and mix thoroughly. Add sesame seeds on top, and serve.

Alkaline Foods You Should Include in Your Daily Diet

If you have paid close attention to your chemistry lessons during school, you will be familiar with the concept of acid and alkali. If not, then here's a quick brush up: Acids are basically aqueous solutions that have a pH level of less than 7.0 whereas alkalis have a pH level of more than 7.0, water being the neutral component with a pH of 7.0. In simpler terms, acids are sour in taste and corrosive in nature, whereas alkalis are elements that neutralise acids.

During the process of digestion, our stomach secretes gastric acids, which help in breaking down food. The stomach has a pH balance which ranges from 2.0 to 3.5, which is highly acidic but necessary for the process of digestion. However, sometimes, due to unhealthy lifestyle and food habits, the acidic level in the body goes haywire, leading to acidity, acid refluxes and other gastric ailments. If you review the daily diet of most urban dwellers, it contains large amounts of acidic foods such as burger, samosa, pizza, rolls, cheese sandwiches, sausages, bacon, kebabs, colas, doughnuts, pastries, etc - which in the long run can hamper the acidic balance in the stomach. These foods when broken down leaves behind residues that are referred to as acid ash, the main cause of your tummy troubles.Ingredients that are acidic in nature when digested by the body are meats, dairy products, eggs, certain whole grains, refined sugars and processed food items. It is important to note that an ingredient's acid or alkaline forming tendency in the body has nothing to do with the actual pH of the food itself. Citrus fruits are acidic in nature, but citric acid actually has an alkalising effect in our body.

Alkaline foods are important so as to bring about a balance. Like all experts and doctors have been saying for years, we should have a balanced meal with a good mix of everything, rather than restraining ourselves to have only a certain category of food items. Alkaline foods therefore help in countering the risks of acidity and acid refluxes, bringing some sort of relief. Most traditional Indian meals contain alkaline food items to create a balanced diet. If you have ever tried a typical Assamese lunch, it always starts with a dish called Khar. Khar also refers to the main ingredient in the dish, which is an alkali extracted from the peels of a banana varietal known as Bhim Kol. The peels are dry roasted and preserved, and before preparing the dish, are soaked in warm water to obtain a brownish filtrate which is then used in cooking. The dish can be made with different ingredients, but the one made with raw papaya is most cherished, known as Amitar Khar. If raw papaya isn't available then cabbage or squash is used as well. Sometimes, a fried fish head is scrambled into the dish during the later stages of the cooking process. Khar is believed to be good for the stomach, easing digestion.

Alkaline Foods for Your Daily Diet

If you have been indulging in excessive red meat, processed and junk food, it's about time you included some alkaline food in your diet. Here's a list to get you started -

1. Green Leafy Vegetables

Most green leafy vegetables are said to have an alkaline effect in our system. It is not without reason that our elders and health experts always advise us to include greens in our daily diet. They contain essential minerals which are necessary for the body to carry out various functions. Try including spinach, lettuce, kale, celery, parsley, argula and mustard greens in your meals.

2. Cauliflower and Broccoli

If you love sautéed broccoli in Asian spices or gobi matar, they are both good for you. They contain several phytochemicals that are essential for your body. Toss it up with other veggies like capsicum, beans and green peas and you have your health dose right there.

3. Citrus Fruits

Contrary to the belief that citrus fruits are highly acidic and would have an acidic effect on the body, they are the best source of alkaline foods. Lemon, lime and oranges are loaded with Vitamin C and are known to help in detoxifying the system, including providing relief from acidity and heart burn.

4. Seaweed and Sea Salt

Did you know that seaweed or sea vegetables have 10-12 times more mineral content than those grown on land? They are also considered to be highly alkaline food sources and are known to bring about various benefits to the body system. You can tip in nori or kelp into your bowl of soup or stir-fries or make sushi at home. Or just sprinkle some sea salt into your salads, soups, omelette, etc.

5. Root Vegetables

Root vegetables like sweet potato, taro root, lotus root, beets and carrots are great sources of alkali. They taste best when roasted with a little sprinkling of spices and other seasonings. Most often, they are overcooked which makes them lose out all their goodness. Pay attention while cooking and you will fall in love with root veggies as you learn to include them in soups, stir-fries, salads and more.

beetroot6. Seasonal FruitsEvery nutritionist and health expert will tell you that adding seasonal fruits in your daily diet can prove to be beneficial to your health. They come packed with vitamins, minerals and antioxidants that take care of various functions in the body. They are good alkaline food sources too, especially kiwi, pineapple, persimmon, nectarine, watermelon, grapefruit, apricots and apples.

7. Nuts

Love to munch on nuts when hunger pangs kick in? Besides being sources of good fats, they also produce an alkaline effect in the body. However, since they are high in calories, it is important to have limited □uantities of nuts. Include cashews, chestnuts and almonds in your daily meal plan.

8. Onion, Garlic and Ginger

Among the most important ingredients in Indian cooking, onion, garlic and ginger are great flavour enhancers too. You can use them in numerous other ways - garlic to spruce up your morning toast, grated ginger in your soup or tea, freshly sliced onions in salads, etc.

Now that you have this list of alkaline food sources, try and include them in your diet to make the most of their incredible benefit.

Chapter Four

The Alkaline Diet Myth

The alkaline diet is also known as the acid-alkaline diet or the alkaline ash diet. It is based around the idea that the foods you eat leave behind an "ash" residue after they have been metabolized. This ash can be acid or alkaline.

Proponents of this diet claim that certain foods can affect the acidity and alkalinity of bodily fluids, including urine and blood. If you eat foods with an acidic ash, they make the body acidic. If you eat foods with an alkaline ash, they make the body alkaline.

Acid ash is thought to make you vulnerable to diseases such as cancer, osteoporosis, and muscle wasting, whereas alkaline ash is considered to be protective. To make sure you stay alkaline, it is recommended that you keep track of your urine using handy pH test strips.

For those who do not fully understand human physiology and are not nutrition experts, diet claims like this sounds rather convincing. However, is it really true? The following will debunk this myth and clear up some confusion regarding the alkaline diet.

But first, it is necessary to understand the meaning of the pH value. Put simply, the pH value is a measure of how acidic or alkaline something is. The pH value ranges from 0 to 14.

0-7 is acidic

7 is neutral

7-14 is alkaline

For example, the stomach is loaded with highly acidic hydrochloric acid, a pH value between 2 and 3.5. The acidity helps kill germs and break down food.

On the other hand, the human blood is always slightly alkaline, with a pH of between 7.35 to 7.45. Normally, the body has several effective mechanisms (discussed later) to keep the blood pH within this range. Falling out of it is very serious and can be fatal.

Effects Of Foods On Urine And Blood pH

Foods leave behind an acid or alkaline ash. Acid ash contains phosphate and sulfur. Alkaline ash contains calcium, magnesium, and potassium. Certain food groups are considered acidic, neutral, or alkaline.

Acidic: Meats, fish, dairy, eggs, grains, and alcohol.

Neutral: Fats, starches, and sugars.

Alkaline: Fruits, vegetables, nuts, and legumes.

Urine pH

Foods you eat change the pH of your urine. If you have a green smoothie for breakfast, your urine, in a few hours, will be more alkaline than if you had bacon and eggs.

For someone on an alkaline diet, urine pH can be very easily monitored and may even provide instant gratification. Unfortunately, urine pH is neither a good indicator of the overall pH of the body, nor is it a good indicator of general health.

Blood pH

Foods you eat do not change your blood pH. When you eat something with an acid ash like protein, the acids produced are quickly neutralized by bicarbonate ions in the blood. This reaction produces carbon dioxide, which is exhaled through the lungs, and salts, which are excreted by the kidneys in your urine.

During the process of excretion, the kidneys produce new bicarbonate ions, which are returned to the blood to replace the bicarbonate that was initially used to neutralize the acid. This creates a sustainable cycle in which the body is able to maintain the pH of the blood within a tight range.

Therefore, as long as your kidneys are functioning normally, your blood pH will not be influenced by the foods you eat, whether they are acidic or alkaline. The claim that eating alkaline foods will make your body or blood pH more alkaline is not true.

Acidic Diet And Cancer

Those who advocate an alkaline diet claim that it can cure cancer because cancer can only grow in an acidic environment. By eating an alkaline diet, cancer cells cannot grow but die.

This hypothesis is very flawed. Cancer is perfectly capable of growing in an alkaline environment. In fact, cancer grows in normal body tissue which has a slightly alkaline pH of 7.4. Many experiments have confirmed this by successfully growing cancer cells in an alkaline environment.

However, cancer cells do grow faster with acidity. Once a tumor starts to develop, it creates its own acidic environment by breaking down glucose and reducing circulation. Therefore, it is not the acidic environment that causes cancer but the cancer that causes the acidic environment.

Even more interesting is a 2005 study by the National Cancer Institute which uses vitamin C (ascorbic acid) to treat cancer. They found that by administering pharmacologic doses intravenously, ascorbic acid successfully killed cancer cells without harming normal cells. This is another example of cancer cells being vulnerable to acidity, as opposed to alkalinity.

In short, there is no scientific link between eating an acidic diet and cancer. Cancer cells can grow in both acidic and alkaline environments.

Acidic Diet And Osteoporosis

Osteoporosis is a progressive bone disease characterized by a decrease in bone mineral content, leading to lowered bone density and strength and higher risk of a broken bone.

Proponents of the alkaline diet believe that in order to maintain a constant blood pH, the body takes alkaline minerals like calcium from the bones to neutralize the acids from an acidic diet. As discussed above, this is absolutely not true. The kidneys and the respiratory system are responsible for regulating blood pH, not the bones.

In fact, many studies have shown that increasing animal protein intake is positive for bone metabolism as it increases calcium retention and activates IGF-1 (insulin-like growth factor-1) that stimulates bone regeneration. Thus, the hypothesis that an acidic diet causes bone loss is not supported by science.

Acidic Diet And Muscle Wasting

Advocates of the alkaline diet believe that in order to eliminate excess acid caused by an acidic diet, the kidneys will steal amino acids (building blocks of protein) from muscle tissues, leading to muscle loss. The proposed mechanism is similar to the one causing osteoporosis.

As discussed, blood pH is regulated by the kidneys and the lungs, not the muscles. Hence, acidic foods like meats, dairy, and eggs do not cause muscle loss. As a matter of fact, they are complete dietary proteins that will support muscle repair and help prevent muscle wasting.

What Did Our Ancestors Eat?

A number of studies have examined whether our pre-agricultural ancestors ate net acidic or net alkaline diets. Very interestingly, they found that about half of the hunter-gatherers ate net acid-forming diets, while the other half ate net alkaline-forming diets.

Acid-forming diets were more common as people moved further north of the equator. The less hospitable the environment, the more animal proteins they ate. In more tropical environments where fruits and vegetables were abundant, their diet became more alkaline.

From an evolutionary perspective, the theory that acidic or protein-rich diets cause diseases like cancer, osteoporosis, and muscle loss is not valid. Half of the hunter-gatherers were eating net acid-forming diets, yet, they had no evidence of such degenerative diseases.

It is worth noting that there is no one-size-fits-all diet that works for everyone, which is why Metabolic Typing is so helpful in determining your optimal diet. Due to our genetic variances, some people will benefit from an acidic diet, some an alkaline diet, and some in between. Thus the saying: one man's food can be another man's poison.

It is true that many people who have switched to an alkaline diet see significant health improvements. However, do bear in mind that other reasons may be at work:

Most of us do not eat enough vegetables and fruits. According to the Center for Disease and Prevention, only 9% of Americans eat enough vegetables and 13% enough fruits. If you switch to an alkaline diet, you are automatically eating more vegetables and fruits. After all, they are very rich in phytochemicals, antioxidants, and fiber which are essential to good health. When you eat more vegetables and fruits, you are probably eating less processed foods too.

Eating less dairy and eggs will benefit those who are lactose-intolerant or have a food sensitivity to eggs, which is rather common among the general population.

Eating less grains will benefit those who are gluten-sensitive or have leaky gut or an autoimmune disease.

Alkaline Water

One last point worth mentioning is that many people believe that drinking alkaline water (pH of 9.5 vs. pure water's pH of 7.0.) is healthier based on similar reasoning as the alkaline diet. Anyhow, it is not true. Water that is too alkaline can be detrimental to your health and lead to nutritional disequilibrium.

If you drink alkaline water all the time, it will neutralize your stomach acid and raise the alkalinity of your stomach. Over time, it will impair your ability to digest food and absorb nutrients and minerals. With less acidity in the stomach, it will also open the door for bacteria and parasites to get into your small intestine.

The bottom line is that alkaline water is not the answer to good health. Do not be fooled by marketing gimmicks. Instead, invest in a good water filtration system for your home. Clean, filtered water is still the best water for your body.

Chapter Five

Benefits of Alkaline Diet for Diabetics

The human body is, to some degree, alkaline by design. By maintaining it alkaline we allow it to run at an ideal level. Nevertheless, millions of reactions of our metabolism yield acidic wastes as end products. When we consume an excessive amount of acid-producing foods and not enough alkaline-forming foods we aggravate the body acid intoxication. If we let these acid-wastes build-up throughout the body, a disorder known as acidosis develops over time.

Acidosis will progressively debilitate our body vital functions, if we do not quickly take corrective actions. Acidosis, or body over-acidity, is in fact one of the leading causes of human aging. It makes our body highly vulnerable to the series of the deadly degenerative chronic diseases, such as diabetes, cancer, arthritis, as well as heart diseases.

For this reason, the biggest challenge we humans have to face to protect our lives is actually to find the right way to reduce the production, and to maximize the elimination of the body acidic wastes. To avoid acidosis and the age-related diseases, and to continue running at its highest level possible, our body needs a healthy lifestyle. This lifestyle should include regular exercises, a balanced nutrition, a clean physical environment, and a way of living that brings the lowest stress possible. A healthy lifestyle allows our body to keep its acid waste content at the lowest level possible.

The alkaline diet, also known as the pH miracle diet, seems to fit the best the design of the human body. This is mainly because it helps neutralize the acid wastes and allows flushing them out from the body. People should look at alkaline diet as general dietary boundaries for humans to abide by. The persons who have particular health issues and special medical diets might better accommodate those diets to alkaline diet boundaries.

Alkaline Diet Benefits for Diabetics

The miracle alkaline diet will help improve the overall health of the persons suffering from diabetes. As it does for other human beings, alkaline diet will help boost their body physiology and metabolism, as well as their immune system. This diet will allow diabetics to have a better control on their blood sugar. It is also going to help not only in reducing their weight gain and the risks of cardiovascular diseases, but also in keeping their cholesterol level low.

In fact, the alkaline diet allows a better management of diabetes and, as a result, it helps diabetics avoid more easily the degenerative diseases connected to their condition. So by following an alkaline diet, despite their health situation, diabetics can, at the same time, live healthier and extend considerably their life expectancy.

Diabetics Acid-Alkaline Food Details

In general, people who want to follow an alkaline diet need to select their daily food items from an 'Acid-Alkaline Foods Chart'. We recently published a 'Diabetics Acid-Alkaline Food Chart'. The use of this specific chart allows diabetics to conform to both the alkaline diet rule and the glycemic index rule.

The alkaline diet rule sets general nutritional guidelines. According to this diet plan, our daily food intake should be composed of a minimum of 80 percent of alkaline-forming foods, and of no more than 20 percent of acidifying food products. Additionally, the diet highlights that the more alkaline a food item is, the better it is actually; and on the other hand the more acidifying a food product is, the worse it should be for the human body.

As for the glycemic index rule, it divides foods into four main categories with respect to their ability to raise the blood sugar. This ability is now measured by the glycemic index GI that ranges from 0 to 100. Foods that contain almost no carbohydrates and that have, in conse☐uence, a negligible glycemic index (GI~0); diabetics may take them freely. Foods containing carbohydrates with a low glycemic index (GI 55 or less); people with diabetes should eat these products with some precaution. Foods that have carbohydrates of high glycemic index (GI 56 or more); diabetics must, so far as possible, exclude them from their diet. Processed foods; diabetics will need to consult the manufacturers' labels to figure out their particular glycemic index values.

You can find more details on the glycemic index of foods on the web, at the following locations: the University of Sydney and the American Diabetes Association.

Diabetics Top Best and Top Worst Foods

Intended for the people affected by diabetes, the 'Diabetics Acid-Alkaline Food Chart' divides foods into six categories. The list below goes from the top best to the top worst foods.

1. Alkalizing food items with GI~0. They are among the top best foods. Diabetics may eat them freely.

Asparagus; broccoli; parsley; celery; lettuce; carob; vegetable juices; mushrooms; s□uash; okra; zucchini; cauliflower; garlic/onions; green beans; beets; cabbage; raw spinach; lemons; avocados; limes; goat cheese; herb teas; stevia; lemon water;

ginger tea; green tea; canola oil; olive oil; flax-seed oil.

2. Alkalizing food products that have a GI of 55 or less. People who have diabetes should take them with moderation, because of their glycemic index.

Barley grass; sweet potato; carrots; fresh corn; olives; peas/soybeans; tomatoes; bananas; cherries; pears; oranges; peaches; grapefruit; mangoes; kiwi; papayas; berries; apples; almonds; Brazil nut; wild rice; chestnuts; coconut; ◻uinoa; hazelnuts; lentils; soy milk; soy cheese; goat milk; breast milk; raw honey; whey.

3. Acidifying foods with a GI~0. Diabetics should consume them with caution, being their acid-producing character.

Rhubarb; cooked spinach; pork; shellfish; liver; oysters; beef; venison; lamb; cold water fish; chicken; turkey; eggs; butter; buttermilk; cottage cheese; cheese; corn oil; lard; margarine; sunflower oil; wine; beer; coffee; cocoa; tea; mayonnaise; molasses; mustard; vinegar; artificial sweeteners.

4. Acidifying foods having a GI of 55 or less. Considering both their acid-forming feature and

their glycemic index, people with diabetes will need to eat them with restraint.

Lima beans; navy beans; kidney beans; pinto beans; blueberries; cranberries; sour cherries; prunes; plums; brown rice; sprouted wheat bread; corn; oats/rye; whole wheat/rye bread; pasta/pastries; wheat; walnuts; peanuts; pistachios; cashews; pecans; sunflower seeds; sesame; yogurt; cream; raw milk; custard; homogenized milk; ice cream; chocolate.

5. Alkaline-forming foods with a GI of 56 or more. Because of their high glycemic index, these products are among the worst foods for diabetics. Therefore, people who suffer from diabetes need to avoid them.

Turnip; beetroot; tofu; potato with skins; figs; grapes/raisins; dates; melons; pineapple; watermelon; rice syrup; maple syrup; raw sugar; amaranth; millet.

6. Acid-producing foods with a GI of 56 or more. These items are too acidic and have too high-glycemic index carbohydrates. They represent the top worst foods for diabetics. Thus, diabetes sufferers need to cut them completely from their meals.

Chapter Six

Acid to Alkaline Diet, How to Lose Weight and Live a Healthier Lifestyle Naturally

The acid to alkaline diet is becoming a more talked about subject nowadays but still the majority of the population are unaware of what it is. People who die young, have health problems, suffer from obesity etc., generally have a very acidic internal environment whereas people who live to a very old age and don't suffer from serious health problems have an internal environment that is more alkaline in nature.

In the modern Western world the vast majority of people live a very unhealthy lifestyle, predominantly eating junk and unhealthy food and being constantly exposed to other factors that drastically impact our health in a negative way, in drastic contrast to the acid to alkaline diet. According to the World Health Organization (WHO), there are more that one billion obese adults world-wide, with around 300 million of them clinically obese. This statistic is scary and is dramatically increasing everyday!

In order for us to live a healthy life, we must not be over weight, avoid serious disease and illnesses and generally live to a good old age with vitality and vigour, it is essential that we pay attention to the acid to alkaline diet. By observing your bodies pH levels and eating accordingly to ensure your body is more alkaline than acidic, people experience things like rapid weight loss (by an accelerated fat disposal process), they will live longer, feel less stressed, have an improved immune system, get better and more restful sleep, have more energy and can also experience an increase in libido. These benefits alone are of course of tremendous importance to health, longevity and a happy life. By allowing the body to detox in this way through the acid to alkaline diet people also have an increased ability to absorb vitamins and minerals and help avoid many nasty diseases including cancer and arthritis. With a more alkaline body, stress and pressure on the internal organs is eased, skin, bones and cells regenerate and help keep you youthful.

Conversely, if a person's body is too acidic they can easily experience obesity by gaining and holding onto fat, they will age quicker, a lack of energy will be common, they will easily and consistently attract disease and virus' and create an internal environment where yeast and bacteria can easily thrive.

The majority of people living in the Western world don't follow an acid to alkaline diet and are generally more on the acidic scale. This is due largely to our diet. Eating things like junk food, burgers, fizzy drinks, having a high sugar intake, fried foods, unnatural fruit juices, imitation foods, energy drinks and processed foods for example, all push our bodies internal environment down on the acidic scale. There are even some otherwise healthy foods to be aware of, strawberries, mangos and peaches for example are very high in sugar, therefore create an acidic environment in the body. Some other surprises that also cause acidic build up include rice, tuna, oats and cheese, so these foods are to be limited when following an acid to alkaline diet. This is one reason why it is very important to know exactly what foods will cause an acid reaction and which will make you more alkaline. Other considerations that also cause our bodies to be more acidic include various chemicals, tobacco, radiation, pesticides, artificial sweeteners, air pollution, alcohol, drugs and stress.

Optimal pH to get all the benefits from alkalinity is 7.4pH. If your body goes 3-4 points either way you will die! The pH scale is as follows:

- ✓ 0 = *total acid/battery acid, hydrochloric acid*
- ✓ 1 = *gastric juices*
- ✓ 2 = *vinegar*
- ✓ 3 = *beer*
- ✓ 4 = *wine, tomato juice*
- ✓ 5 = *rain*
- ✓ 6 = *milk*
- ✓ 7 = *pure water*
- ✓ 8 = *sea water*
- ✓ 9 = *baking soda*
- ✓ 10 = *detergent, milk of magnesia*
- ✓ 11 = *ammonia, lime water*
- ✓ 12 = *bleach*

✓ *13 = lye*
✓ *14 = Total Alkaline/Sodium Hydroxide*

The acid to alkaline diet will help your body stay at the optimal range, around 7.4pH. The bodies reaction to trying to keep this acid, alkaline balance is both incredible and fascinating. When your body is too acidic it tries everything to get to a more alkaline state. When this happens the body stores some acid in your fat to keep it from doing harm to our body which is a good thing, but your body then holds on to the fat for protection, causing the person to put on weight.

When there is excess acid internally, the body finds alkaline elsewhere from your bones and teeth but your bones and teeth get so drained that they become frail and start to decay. This can lead to many diseases of the bones and teeth including arthritis and tooth decay. This would not happen if a person were following an acid to alkaline diet.

The build up of acid generally will settle away from your healthier organs but instead it gravitates towards your weakest organs that are already prone to disease. It's like a pack of wolves looking for the weakest amongst the herd, picking off the easy prey. As your weaker organs are targeted it makes it much easier for serious diseases to set in, including cancer. It is important to realise that cancer cells become dormant if you are at 7.4pH (which is the bodies optimum pH levels), thus further underlining the importance of maintaining a healthy pH level in our bodies by following the acid to alkaline diet.

When there is acid in the system it also contaminates your blood stream. This in turn prevents the bloods ability to deliver oxygen to the tissues. RBC's are surrounded by a negative charge so they can bounce off each other and move around in the blood very ⬜uickly and deliver their goodness.

But when you are too acidic they lose their negative charge and they stick together, causing them to move very slowly. This causes them to struggle to deliver nutrients and oxygen in our system. One of the first symptoms of this poisoning is you start to feel a loss of energy even though you are getting enough sleep. Starting an acid to alkaline diet can correct this very ⬜uickly. Your blood also has this reaction after drinking alcohol.

Let's put all this into perspective; it takes about 33 glasses of water to neutralize one glass of coke! I'm not even going to mention here what it takes to neutralize some of the other things that we are putting into our bodies, I think you get the picture!

One great way to consistently make your body more alkaline is by having green drinks everyday. They are very easy to make, taste great and are packed with vitamins, minerals and chlorophyll which fuel our body. Chlorophyll is a big part of the acid to alkaline diet and is the green blood of plants. It is a very powerful detoxify-er, blood builder, cleaner and oxygen booster. In fact, the benefits of chlorophyll on our bodies are far too numerous to include in this article. There are many recipes for making tasty green drinks.

Tips To Transition To Alkaline Eating

Have you ever been in a swimming pool where the levels of chlorine were out of whack? It stings your eyes and makes them all itchy and red. That's because the pH levels were not neutral. A similar thing is actually going on inside our bodies if our pH levels are also unbalanced. When our body is more acidic than alkaline on the pH scale, we suffer health problems.

Why? Well, acidic blood is toxic to your cells, which can't do their job of fighting bacteria if they are damaged. Also, damaged cells carry less life-giving oxygen around the body. And less oxygen means less energy, which can lead to more health issues. It's all pretty depressing, isn't it? Luckily we can fix this unbalanced and dangerous situation in a quick, easy, and remarkably cheap way.

First, you need to reduce the things in your life that are making you acidic. Probably the number one non-food way the body becomes acidic is emotional stress. If your life is go-go-go, then it's vital that you put mindfulness, meditation, and gentle exercise on your daily agenda. That feeling of calm you get after having a long hot bath or writing in your journal is helping both your mind AND your body.

Second, a few □uick changes to your diet will help you to fight inflamed cells by becoming alkaline. Here are my seven secrets to transition to alkaline eating:

1. Start drinking lemon water.

Once in the body lemon becomes alkaline. So drop a lemon slice into your water for a wonderful pick-me-up drink that'll keep you hydrated and help detoxify your liver. Try and choose filtered water and if possible invest in an alkalizing water filtration system.

2. Get to know the acid/alkaline chart.

Print out the chart I've included and stick it on your fridge for easy reference. Start by focusing on eating the foods on the "alkaline" list. Here's a mini-challenge: Try adding one new alkaline food to either breakfast, lunch, or dinner each day for two weeks.

3. De-clutter your kitchen.

Begin with your shopping lists and clean out your fridge and pantry of all processed junk foods, foods that are sabotaging your weight loss. Remember, out of sight, out of mind!

4. Invest in a blender.

Having the right equipment to quickly whip up a high-nutrition smoothie makes everything so much easier. Keep it on the counter ready to go, not hiding in the cabinet!

5. Find one alkaline smoothie recipe that you like.

It sometimes takes a few tries before you find the perfect smoothie combination. Here is one of my favorite alkaline smoothie recipes, which tastes great and alkalizes you fast:

Emily's Energizer: ½ stick celery, handful of spinach leaves, handful of kale leaves, a handful of fresh pineapple chunks (or mango), ½ frozen banana, 3 or 4 sprigs of parsley, a sprinkle of chia seeds, a squeeze of lemon, a scoop of certified organic pea protein powder, 1 cup of coconut water, and ice.

6. Focus on eating something green at every meal.

A really simple rule of thumb is to make sure every meal (yes, including breakfast!) has something green on the plate: smoothies with some leaves and vegetables for breakfast, quinoa and steamed veggie salads for lunch, veggie and lentil soups for dinner, or fresh fish or organic chicken with salad or vegetables. Oh, and don't forget the snack either. Try slicing up a carrot, a Lebanese cucumber, and a few sticks of celery so you can snack on yummy hummus guilt-free.

7. Plan your meals on Sunday.

Every Sunday I focus on early preparation for the upcoming week. Not only does it mean I avoid temptation foods and self-sabotage, but I feel more calm knowing that my meals for the week are sorted. Organizing your meals for the week is the most important thing you can do to take control of your body, health, and weight. I always spend Sundays at the farmers market and spend a couple of hours in the kitchen, then I'm set for the week.

Conclusion

If you have heard of the Atkins diet, then the Acid Alkaline Diet is the complete opposite of that. The Atkins diet is a high protein, high fat but low carbohydrates diet. But such diets have a tendency to leave one low on energy and also they seem to be improper gastronomically speaking. An acid alkaline diet on the other hand is not only useful for weight loss but over an above that is extremely beneficial to the body functioning. An Acid alkaline, also known as an alkaline ash diet, alkaline acid diet and the alkaline diet, keeps the ph level of the body balanced and so safeguards against various illnesses. Even chronic diseases like arthritis can be not only prevented but also cured if such a diet is followed.

The basis of a diet that is acid alkaline lies in the fact that our body ph ideally should be a 7.3. This slightly alkaline level of the body ph keeps all the vital organs functioning well, as well as the absorption of various minerals is optimized. When this ph tilts to the acidic side trouble starts brewing. An acidic ph level leads to almost all body parts suffering in one way or the other. Now since our body needs to be alkaline in nature it should reflect in our food intake too. Foods that are alkalizing should be consumed mush more as opposed to the acidifying foods. Translated in a simpler language this would mean more of vegetable and fruit consumption and very low meats and oil intake. If the body's alkaline minerals such as calcium, magnesium and potassium levels drop so will its health causing it to degenerate and its defenses to drop guard. An alkaline diet protects that from happening. An acid alkaline or an alkaline ash diet comprises of 80% alkalizing foods and 20 % acidic foods. Since the acid alkaline ratio in the body should be one is to four our food intake should be of similar nature.

An alkaline diet is not only recommended to shed those extra pounds but is also and more importantly a great means of regaining lost health and leading a longer and more diseases free life. This diet is especially recommended to those who feel tired most of the time. Stress and a low energy level can both be done away with a diet that is acid alkaline. Those who suffer from frequent viral fevers or those who have a nasal congestion most of the time can lead healthier lives if they have a diet that is acid alkaline. Weak nails, dryness, headaches, muscle pain, hives, joint pains, and many more such diseases find their answer in an alkaline ash diet.

A higher level of vegetable intake is recommended in an alkaline ash diet. Lemons should be s□ueezed into water drinks. Millet or □uinoa is preferred over wheat, olive oil over vegetable oil and soups like miso are very useful for following an alkaline ash diet.

Lost health and vigor can be regained and many chronic illnesses prevented as well as cured if an acid alkaline diet is followed. It is a fairly easy diet plan, which should adapt for a longer and healthier life span.

www.ingramcontent.com/pod-product-compliance
Lightning Source LLC
Chambersburg PA
CBHW060104300526
45788CB00015B/1521